Game Over, MS

Heather Collins-Grattan Floyd

DEDICATION

To my wonderful family: My husband, Kevin Floyd;
my parents, the Rev. Robert and Ann Collins;
my sister, Heidi Collins;
my in-laws, Gene and Carol Lempicki,
and Mary Floyd;
and our pit-bull and bichon frisé,
Jigsaw and Ketchup.

CONTENTS

ACKNOWLEDGEMENTS

In addition to the people mentioned in the Dedication and my extended family, I have a lot of people to thank for their support and encouragement over these years. Special thanks to Joe and Lori Christiano, Herman and Sharron Bailey, Steve Bond, Cynthia Aden, Diane Keely, Maureen McDermott Cannon, Misha Kaura, Emily Wojcik, Eileen Friedman, Lorraine Cox Dora, Donna Reeves Page, Nicole Spivey Jhonson, Darlene Demko, Christine Sawyer Driscoll, Tim Cerio, Scott McClelland, Aki Aoyama, Christopher Cooper, Steve and Lori Leveen, Annette Britton, Beate Buchholz-Allen, Susan Granick, Diane Southards, Ben Dicks, Kristi Meeks, Brenda Sokolowski, Nick and Mary Hall, Caryn Forrest, Beth York, Kaci Bloemers, Adam Kaufman, Sandy Kelley, Ann-Marie Jaglal, Rachele Scholes, Carol Jaeger, Celeste Simon, Herme de Wyman Miro, Marie Hope Davis, Helene Starr, Dr. William McKeen, Victor and Barbara Brizel, Linda Catalano, David Broughton, Charles Smith, Don Alducin, Ed Crawford, Genene Hirschhorn, Melissa Vanefsky, Lita Small, Elise Doline, Laura Gafford Alonso, Tom Judson, Darren Preston Lane, Scott McClelland, Dr. Marc H. Feinberg, Dr. Randy Katz, Dr. Adrian Lavina, Dr. Christina Curran, Dr. Melissa Carlson, Dr. Douglas Rolfe, Newsmax, Brian Mudd, the extended Grattan family, and, of course, John Shuff.

FOREWORD

BY JOHN SHUFF

A Chinese proverb says, "The journey of a thousand miles starts with a single step."

Let me back you up to 1975. At the time I thought I had it made. Great family, super job as the Chief Financial Officer of a prestigious Fortune 500 Company, financial security. You name it. Nothing was going to stop me. Absolutely nothing.

Well not so fast, John – there was one thing and its ugly name was multiple sclerosis, which

I had been diagnosed with that year at the Mayo Clinic. After only two days of tests, Dr. Raul Espinosa looked me in the eye and quietly said, "You are a classic Sclerotic."

It's said that big boys don't cry. When it sunk in that I had an incurable disease, I did. My wife, Margaret Mary, was five-hundred miles away at our home in Belleville, Illinois. When I told her the doctor's diagnosis, the line was silent – and then interrupted by tears – tears of fear, fear of the unknown and our uncertain future. With a four-year-old and a newborn, our life became undeniably more complicated.

Like many I denied having the disease, until in 1980 when I collapsed in front of my wife on the driving range at our club in Greenwich, Connecticut. At that moment my life and that of my family's changed forever. I was to never walk again, in addition to the other complications that are a part of the MS surprise package.

My journey of a thousand miles began in September, 1980, and is still in progress some 38 years later.

You've heard the old saying "Crawl before you walk." I had to do just that, because neurologically I couldn't perform this simple movement. It was a signal to the neurologists that I had a significant neurological deficit. I now know what babies encounter, except I was 40.

I also learned the meaning of something my dad routinely said to his three boys, "I cried because I had no shoes, until I met a man who had no feet." I never considered the implications of this until I rehabbed side-by-side with people with strokes, kids with cerebral palsy, and teenagers with devastating head injury cases.

For the first time in my life I realized what bad really was. I intuitively relate to my dad's admonition and have never complained about my condition. I've vowed to God that I'll take whatever is dished out, knowing that someone is always worse off than me.

Permit me to share with you a story about John Shuff that I'm not proud of. In 1973 I was appointed by the Governor of Illinois to the Bi-State Commission, a group of people from Illinois and Missouri in charge of mass transportation in the metropolitan St. Louis area. As a member of this body I voted against a proposition in 1974 to adapt some buses in our jurisdiction for the disabled.

I relate this story to you because in voting against this proposition for lack of definitive cost benefits, I deprived the disabled of HOPE. For some HOPE of going to work, visiting a family member, HOPE of wanting to be normal, to get back in the hunt.

Today, I'm embarrassed and disgusted at the lack of sensitivity toward a group that I've now joined. I confess this to you to seek absolution for this grievous error in judgment to ask that you deprive no one of HOPE. If you don't realize it, "HOPE" is the sustenance we live on. The word is part of our daily vocabulary – I HOPE it doesn't rain, I HOPE she likes this present, etc.

I never dreamed that one day I would be disabled and would need an environment that would accommodate me and my sidekick, my wheelchair. Ironically, I now "HOPE" that everywhere I go I'll find accessibility.

DEPRIVE NO ONE OF HOPE, IT MIGHT BE ALL THEY HAVE. WITHOUT IT WE DIE INSIDE FROM THE LACK OF HOPE'S NOURISHMENT.

This reminds me of another lesson that having a chronic illness has taught me. In 1987 I gave a talk to foreign priests and nuns at The Catholic Theological Union in Chicago. The subject of the symposium was Human Suffering. I chose the theme "Fear versus Lack of

Knowledge" because fear is a part in our lives. For many fear is consuming, overwhelming. So, I posited the question:

"IF GOD WERE TO COME INTO THIS ROOM AND LOOK EACH ONE OF US IN THE EYE AND TELL US WHAT WAS IN STORE FOR US FOR THE REST OF OUR LIFE, WHAT WOULD BE YOUR REACTION?"

The idea shocked and surprised them – because for some, the news wouldn't be that good. It would provoke great fear and uncertainty. Instinctively, none of us would know how to cope with this. Our minds would focus on the worst. For many, it would be paralyzing, mind numbing, and downright depressing.

The way I've attempted to overcome the fears created by MS is by understanding it. You do this by obtaining knowledge about the subject you're dealing with. My illness sent shock waves through me and my wife, Margaret

Mary, who has remained by my side during this long (now in its forty-third year of our fifty-five-year marriage) and incomplete journey.

We handle my disability in different ways because of our personalities. But one thing we've both tried to do is understand the implications involved in MS. From temporary blindness in my right eye, to the loss of bodily functions, to paralysis, to slurred speech, to losing my ability to walk and being confined to a wheelchair, MS has had its way with me.

Both of us have attempted to understand what no doctor could predict or understand about the insidious monster that invaded my body. However, our spirit has never dimmed – our undaunted spirit to defeat this monster, to punch it in the face has existed for 43 years. We will never give up; NEVER. To give up HOPE is to die mentally and then permanently.

Margaret Mary read insatiably about MS.

I've tried alternative therapies: snake venom shots, hyperbaric oxygen and acupuncture treatments over long periods of time, and Botox to help my bladder function. I've tried a gluten-free diet but didn't stick with it. I had success with ACTH (adrenocorticotropic hormone), but after three and a half years I began to experience psychotic behavior – no more ACTH.

However, it turned out to be the drug that saved me in 1980 when there was some doubt about me surviving. Biogen's MS drugs Avonex and Tysabri stabilized my condition, but I was advised to cease the Tysabri IV injections to avoid developing brain tumors.

None of this was and is today easy to accept, but by understanding the devil in front of me made it infinitely easier to cope and to fight. Please don't ever let fear overcome you. Instead fight it by truly understanding the problem that confronts you. Believe me, this will give you HOPE and the capacity to formulate a game plan for coping with fear.

It's common to have people refer to me as being a victim of MS. I've learned that victims wait for everything to get better. They wait for tomorrow, a time when they'll start dieting, stop smoking, start exercising. Waiting is for victims. It's for those who can't and don't make things happen.

Action is for VICTORS. VICTORS are change agents. They don't react to change, they create it. VICTORS are motivated by an intense desire to succeed. VICTORS concentrate on finding ways to improve their tomorrow. VICTORS assume responsibility for their happiness. VICTORS improve their tomorrow by realizing that each day things will be better because they want it better.

That's the only way I got myself out of a bed that I was confined to for three years. During those bleak days I developed an intense desire to fight and to show my wife and young children that I wasn't a quitter.

For a moment let me talk about you. When Mother Teresa said, "You can do no great things, only small things with great love," she was referring to you and people like you. Let's hope and pray that cures for MS and other illnesses will be found. And that leads me to another incredibly important factor: prayer. Prayer is something we all need and should engage in every day. Without prayer, there cannot be hope.

I've covered a lot of ground here, talking about hope, fear, victims versus victors, love, and your caring. For 43 years out of our 55-year marriage, my Margaret Mary has lived with the ravages of MS – too private to discuss.

She's stood steadfastly with me when many people have left spouses with MS, she has "for better or for worse, in sickness and in health, until death do us part," being the reason for my determination to get well and to be as normal as

I can for the person I love and respect – what a partner, what a fighter, what an inspiration for all.

However, permit me to share one final thought. A woman I worked closely with in Southern Illinois was Sister Paulette Colling, head of St. Elizabeth's Hospital in Belleville. Before I left to move to New York, she called me into her office and thanked me for my help as her Board chair for the past three years.

She knew I had been diagnosed with MS, and she said something I've never forgotten, and which I hope you won't either. In a gentle voice she said, "Mr. Shuff, please remember, 'Life is not a problem to be solved, but a mystery to be lived.'"

Begin living your mystery today. May God bless you.

CHAPTER 1: THE MS TACKLEBOX: SYSTEMS

I wanted to wait at least 15 years after being diagnosed with multiple sclerosis before writing this book, and it has been 18 years now. I get looks of astonishment when I tell people that I have MS, and I'd like to share with you in these pages how I keep it under control.

There are so many books and articles that advocate one singular fix to MS, usually saying it's best to simply eat a diet that is "natural" or "low-fat" or something that says to me "no fun." And your doctor will likely give you a prescription and tell you it "should help delay" the symptoms.

You don't want to settle for delaying the stupid symptoms. You want to try to stop the MS in its tracks, and eliminate future symptoms and any further hassle, thankyouverymuch. Right?

I figured I wouldn't have any true proof that my multifaceted, total solution works until I'd had success at keeping it at bay for quite a while.

The system I've developed is not a cure to MS, but rather a solution. It doesn't involve special exercises or eating less fat or less sugar, so in my opinion it's the ideal system.

I wrote an article 10 years ago about this system, and I still stick to the same formula as I did back then. Actually, the formula hasn't changed much since I was diagnosed in October 2000, so I've followed this system for 18 years now.

The good people of Newsmax Media published my article about this system on NewsmaxHealth.com on August 26, 2008, and the rest of this chapter is an updated and expanded version of the article:

Defeating MS: From Curse to Blessing

I'm not a doctor – I have no medical training whatsoever. But I am a 37-year-old woman [now 47] who has kept her MS under control for over a dozen years.

One day recently [in summer 2008], I was in the checkout line at Walgreens, and there was a woman sitting in a scooter-chair at the front of the line, paying for her merchandise. She gingerly stood up so she could validate her payment information on the little padscreen, then she sat down again.

Hmm, I thought. *Her legs work just well enough for her to stand up, so her condition isn't caused by full paralysis.* I wondered if she had MS.

As she gathered up the plastic bags with her goods to get ready to roll out the door, the young man in line behind her (and in front of me) asked her if she needed any help. After she declined, he asked the cashier for a pack of cigarettes.

"Oh, I forgot the milk!" exclaimed the woman in the scooter-chair. She turned her head toward the young man behind her and said, "I need my milk just like you need your cigarettes."

Whoa – that solidified it – I was 90% sure she had MS now.

"So, you're a big milk-drinker?" I asked her.

"Yeah," she said.

"Do you have the B blood type?"

"What?"

"Do you have the B blood type?" I repeated, adding, "B positive or B negative?"

"No. [Pause.] Wait – yeah! I do!" she said, incredulous that I'd guessed it correctly.

"So do I. That's also why I have multiple sclerosis." (I know, I know – unabashedly leading the witness.)

"So do I!" she exclaimed. At that moment, I had to hide my excitement over the possibility that I might be able to help this stranger control her condition, or at least help her to be able to understand it more thoroughly.

She looked me up and down, obviously amazed at how healthy I look, and asked me how long ago I was diagnosed. It turned out that she was diagnosed only one year before I was – eight years ago for me (with a warning that I "might have it" four years before that), and nine for her.

I told her about how I've been following the Blood Type Diet™ for over 10 years, and how people have had amazing results by following the diet – and that milk is a very good food for "Type Bs like us."

But it was my lunch hour, and I had to get back to work – so I didn't have time to delve into the details about how the diet's developer, Dr. Peter D'Adamo, points out in his book *Eat Right 4 Your Type* that Type Bs tend to be more susceptible to MS and similar immune-system disorders than are people with the other three blood types (O, A, and AB).

As I fished in my purse for a piece of paper on which to write the name of the diet book for her, I saw the little *Blood Type B Food, Beverage, and Supplement Lists* booklet (a condensed version of the main book) that I keep on hand for reference when dining out at restaurants. *Of course!* I thought.

"In fact, why don't you have this?" I said, and I handed the booklet to her.

"Oh, I can't take that from you!" she said politely. But I insisted, and she accepted it and thanked me.

But the Blood Type Diet is only one part of my overall solution. Let me explain.

The SYSTEMS to Live By

For the purposes of this book, I devised an acronym for the system I use, so the acronym is **SYSTEMS**:

Spirit
Your Mind
Sleep
Temperature
Eat Right
Medicine
Supplements

Let's look at each of these factors and see how they can influence, and hopefully stifle, the process of MS:

<u>S</u>pirit

Find a good house of worship, and attend services every week – even if you don't feel like it or are too tired. (You can take a nap later.) It's the ideal realm in which to foster strength of the mind-body-soul!

You will not only gain spiritual strength, but you'll make friends who will encourage you; you'll realize that your condition is a challenge and a badge of honor, not something to bemoan. Everyone has stories of their own health issues or those of their relatives, and all of that puts it in perspective.

The feedback from others will reinforce the fact that you're not the only one who's going through something. The apostle Paul spoke briefly about his own "thorn in the flesh," and who knows – it might have been MS!

Even if you have disappointing reactions from others (especially from people you thought would have a more mature reaction), it will build character and patience in you. When one of my friends at church found out I was diagnosed with MS, she said, "Oh, I didn't know you were sick."

(Great. So I'm going to be considered "sick" for the rest of my life??)

I don't call MS a sickness, an illness, or a disease. I call it a condition. Words are powerful, and they should be controlled as much as possible.

Incidentally, if I'm asked, "How are you feeeeeling?" I know they're implying pity for my MS. I reply with something like, "I'm doing well! How are *you* feeling?" They're usually taken aback a bit, but that's okay. It's good for all of us to experience how our own words sound!

Your Mind

Even doctors have to be careful not to talk themselves into having the various health conditions of their patients, as too much awareness can make your body actually have sympathy symptoms – whereby your subconscious can cause you to experience what you've been reading or hearing about.

I try to read enough about the latest MS research without spending too much time on it, because I don't want to talk myself into having symptoms that I don't have, or wouldn't have had. The mind is a powerful thing!

Support groups are good for some people, but they're not for everyone. Some people attend support groups just to complain about how terrible their life is and to lament about their latest symptoms, so approach such groups with caution. Rather, I recommend the natural support group of a church instead, because I think the Church is the best support group of them all; and if you don't like one, try another one. Go church-shopping.

Keeping your stress level under control is also incredibly important. Everyone who has MS will tell you that they tend to get exacerbations – or "symptoms" or "flare-ups" or whatever you want to call them – mainly after experiencing a serious stressor in their life. (And it usually occurs after an incident of being too hot, in combination with that stressor.)

Take notice of what exactly makes you feel super-stressed, because it's different for everyone. For me, it's stressors in personal relationships and certain in-person interactions which can cause that awful stress which can bring on an exacerbation – not work-related stress like it is for some people.

This part of the SYSTEMS theory has been tested by fire in my own life. When I was 41 (in 2012), my husband Ron was diagnosed with glioblastoma multiforme, which is the most common and the most lethal form of primary brain cancer.

I knew that this was going to be a very stressful time for me, and I knew I had to stay strong for him and keep him as happy as possible. I resigned from my job to take care of him full-time. My own neurologist, Dr. Marc Feinberg, had previously prescribed Xanax for me to calm my nerves when a relative of mine was going to jail (and I felt intensely stressed about it), so he prescribed Xanax again to help keep my stress levels under control during Ron's illness.

Dr. Feinberg was actually the one who diagnosed Ron with the brain tumor, so he was well aware of what I was dealing with.

With Xanax, the pills are very tiny (and they're not opioids or narcotics), but Dr. Feinberg has always said to cut each one into quarters. So I'd just take one quarter every morning, and that was enough to take the edge off my stress for the day. When it became apparent that Ron's health was severely deteriorating (his personality was becoming more angry, and he wasn't eating much at all), I had to start taking two quarters every morning, because I could feel my stress level building.

Ron's illness only lasted six months before he passed.

I tell this story because you may feel like you're being self-centered when dealing with your own stress that's a reaction to someone else's bad situation. But you'll actually be a more effective human being for others if you take care of yourself so you can stay strong.

I'm not recommending that everyone with MS take Xanax for their occasional stressful days – Xanax can be addictive. Taking a low dose helps to prevent becoming addicted to it. Get your own neurologist's evaluation for whatever stress medication would work best for you, and keep it on hand for use only when you need it. (The Xanax in my medicine cabinet is 6 years old, because I rarely need it.)

Life does bring very stressful events, and some of them make MS seem like child's play. Be ready to tamp it down when your stress level is high, or when you can anticipate the stress.

Sleep

When anyone gets a cold, the body activates the T-cells – which can be "good guys gone bad" if you have MS. When T-cells are activated in someone with MS, these macrophages mistakenly gobble up myelin, which is a protective fatty layer covering everyone's brain and spinal cord. If myelin is gobbled up, it forms scars, or *sclerosis*, in their place.

So if I catch myself coming down with something, I used to take a half-day off to sleep in – and get a really good night's sleep beforehand. Now that I'm in my 40s and have better immunity against colds, if I'm at work, I'll take a nap in my car if I feel myself starting to cough or sneeze more than usual! I set the alarm on my phone for 20 minutes, lock the doors, and put the seat all the way back. Zzzzz.

Even if you're not fighting a cold, sleep and rest are imperative in controlling MS.

If you don't get at least 6.5 hours of sleep at night, it's a good idea to take a 20-minute nap in the afternoon. If you're not a "nap person," be sure to get enough sleep at night. If you can't fall asleep, don't fret! Just be sure to rest. Listen to music you like, or put a show on in the background that you like – and close your eyes.

Remember, don't hesitate to strictly take care of yourself! If you don't, no one will.

Temperature

I live in South Florida, but I always have cold water or soda to drink. If someone with MS is going to be in a hot environment for any length of time, they can drink cold fluids to keep cool on the inside. For reasons still not fully understood, heat can exacerbate MS and its symptoms.

I've noticed while traveling in Pennsylvania and upstate New York during the summer that it's often reeeeally hot indoors! Whereas in South Florida the air-conditioning is always on at full-blast, the cooler northern states tend not to have air-conditioning that's quite as efficient – or perhaps it's just viewed as too expensive and not worth it.

Be sure to speak up, or take control of the thermostat yourself, if your indoor environment is too hot. It's better to be too cold than too hot. No saunas or hot tubs for us! Interestingly, a number of people are diagnosed with MS after being on vacation where they've spent a lot of time in the sauna or hot tub, and they experience sudden unexpected numbness or vision trouble.

Earlier in my career, the company I was working for was going to have a "Fun Day" to have everyone in the marketing and merchandising departments get to know each other better. People who worked in the human resources department handed out sunglasses to us with a sly smile, keeping the details a secret. A rumor was going around that the Fun Day was going to be held all day at an outdoor park.

Ugh. All day at an outdoor park in the South Florida heat, walking around and getting sweaty, and possibly no place to sit down and take a break. No way – that wouldn't work. It would be better to just work all day in the air-conditioned workplace while everyone else had Fun Day. I didn't want to have half of my body go numb again, or lose my vision in one eye for five months again (which I'll tell you about in Chapters 3 and 4).

I emailed the HR department telling them I have MS, and so I couldn't participate in the Fun Day if it was really going to be outdoors. I told them I could have my neurologist give them a letter if necessary. And I told them I would just work all day like usual.

They thanked me for letting them know, and they said I could just take that day off. I was glad that they were so understanding, even though I felt like a wet blanket!

Take care of yourself, and stay cool even if it makes you feel very un-cool! You'll be glad later.

Eat Right

I have strictly followed the Blood Type Diet for 21 years now. Blood types O, A, B, and AB each have certain "healthy" foods and other foods that aren't so healthy, and the theory helps to explain why one person does well on a high-meat, low-grain diet while another person does well on a vegetarian diet. The Blood Type Diet is fully explained and delineated in the book *Eat Right 4 Your Type* by naturopathic physician Dr. Peter D'Adamo.

The science behind the diet has been further solidified in its efficacy by others, including fitness guru and author Joseph "Dr. Joe" Christiano, who is also a certified naturopath. Many nutritionists also advocate this regimen.

Dr. D'Adamo followed in his father's footsteps in researching how each blood type influences an individual's body chemistry – particularly in regards to how well each food is processed in the person's system. He and his father both saw patterns within each of the O, A, B, and AB types; the Rh factor, which is the positive/negative part of your blood type, isn't a factor in the diet.

D'Adamo says in the book that people with the B blood type (like me) tend to fend off cancers better than folks with the other three types, but Type Bs tend to be susceptible to odd autoimmune conditions like MS and lupus.

Sure enough, even though I have dozens of cousins and aunts and uncles, none of them have MS or anything like it. But almost none of them are Type B like I am – they're mostly Type A or AB.

More than half of the people I know who have MS are indeed Type B, even though only about 11% of Americans have that type. However, I know several who are Type A or Type O, and I recommend that everyone consider this diet because it's geared to your own body chemistry.

None of my doctors have pooh-poohed my diet – they'll say, "Keep doing whatever you're doing." They see how healthy I am, and a good doctor wouldn't want to ruin a patient's good health, right? ☺

People of all four types have experienced wonderful health benefits as a result of following this regimen. In case you're wondering, about 48% of Americans are Type O, about 37% are Type A, about 11% are Type B, and about 4% are Type AB.

Beware of the "experts" who belittle this diet. They tend to cite a "lack of evidence" proving that it works. But any study of an overall population in the U.S. will favor tendencies of Type O and/or Type A, which together comprise about 85% of the population.

If you'd like evidence, I cite my 21 years of success as a good start. The fact is that there has not been a large-scale study of whether the Blood Type Diet works or not; this shines a spotlight on the fact that the fields of traditional medicine and alternative medicine don't generally talk to each other. Medical doctors want you to take a medicine, naturopaths want you to follow a natural solution, and I do both.

See how this diet applies to you in the next chapter.

Medicine

I have taken an interferon medication for 18 years now. I was on Avonex for 16 years (a once-a-week injection), and now I've been on Plegridy for the past two years (a once-every-two-weeks injection).

Different people tolerate medicines differently, but there are plenty of options on the market – so if one doesn't work for you, another one will. There have been injectable medicines for MS since 1993, and oral medicines since 2010. We are blessed to live here and now.

I have a great neurologist who's very positive and encouraging, which is incredibly helpful psychologically. Be sure to find a neurologist who is relatable to you, positive, and empowering. Don't entertain any pity-partiers, naysayers, or Debbie Downers. (The neurologist who diagnosed me in 2000, mentioned anonymously in Chapter 3, was all three! But then again, his personality didn't jibe with mine very well, so perhaps that was the problem.)

Make sure you have good chemistry with your neurologist, as odd as that may sound! Don't hesitate to switch to another neurologist who's even in the same practice. It may feel awkward at first, but it'll be worth it to switch. The practice would rather keep you as a patient than lose you to another practice.

When I was diagnosed in 2000, my medicinal options were pretty much "the A-B-C drugs" for MS: Avonex, Betaseron, and Copaxone. But there are now quite a few:

Injectable (Shots)

Daclizumab (Zenapax®, Zinbryta™)

Glatiramer Acetate (Copaxone®, Glatopa®)

Interferon Beta-1a (Avonex®, Rebif®)

Interferon Beta-1b (Extavia®, Betaseron/ Betaferon®)

Peginterferon Beta-1a (Plegridy®)

Oral (Pills)

Azathioprine (Imuran®, Azasan®)

Dimethyl Fumarate (Tecfidera®, BG-12)

Fingolimod (FTY-720, Gilenya®)

Laquinimod

Methotrexate (Trexall®, Matrex®)

Minocycline

Teriflunomide (Aubagio®)

Infusion

Cladribine (Leustat®)

Cyclophosphamide (Cytoxan®)

Gamma Globulin (IVIG)

Mitoxantrone (Novantrone)

Natalizumab (Tysabri®)

Ocrelizumab (Ocrevus™)

Plasmapheresis / Plasma Exchange

Rituximab (Rituxan®)

...One of these medications will work for you. If your doctor is being wishy-washy, get another neurologist.

If you pride yourself on never taking medication, get rid of that pride. You're playing a whole new ballgame – play to win!

Supplements

Folks with MS should not take multivitamins, as these pills have vitamin B-6 and other immune-system–strengthening components; the issue in MS is that the immune system is a bit too strong already, so strengthening it is usually a no-no!

As for me personally, the supplements I take are evening primrose oil (a source of gamma-linolenic acid, which is an omega-6 essential fatty acid), ginkgo biloba, vitamins B-12 and D3, magnesium, and – to help me sleep, but skipping Friday nights to avoid dependence – a very low dose of melatonin. Each individual with MS should try supplements and get their neurologist's input about them first. Be aware of any unusual reactions, such as if ginkgo biloba makes you have any bleeding issues.

If I feel that I'm starting to fight a cold, I drink Emergen-C for one or two days. Emergen-C is a flavored powder you put in a bottle of water. I only drink that if I'm truly trying to prevent a cold, though, because vitamin C can boost the immune system – which is something those of us with MS have to be careful of. It's a delicate balancing act; listen to your body, and don't be quick to take supplement advice from friends or the latest fads.

Incidentally, I do not recommend cannabis. Once you're eating properly per your blood type, you're on an MS medication that works for you, and you're getting into a renewed lifestyle of prioritizing your own health, you'll feel happier and healthier. Many studies have found that marijuana can negatively impact the brain, and the brain is already being impacted in MS. So it's a good idea to avoid things that could be detrimental.

My TSA Snack-Pack Pudding Story

Because swallowing pills can sometimes be awkward or uncomfortable, it's been recommended to me to take pills with either yogurt or pudding, rather than with a liquid. Applesauce also works for some people. Medical professionals have told me that it's easier for your throat to negotiate swallowing a solid with another semi-solid, rather than a solid and a liquid together.

I once went on vacation to visit my Grandma Ruth, so I was flying to Syracuse. I had about a dozen Snack-Pack chocolate puddings (which don't have to be refrigerated) in my carry-on bag for my flight. Well, when going through the TSA check, they stopped me! The guy said that the large amount of pudding was "excessive." I told him I need them to take my pills, and that I have MS.

He discussed it with another TSA official, and they agreed that I could bring them on if I'd agree to a pat-down check. Hey, that was fine with me! So I got patted down by the TSA for my Snack-Packs.

Bottom Line: Prioritize Your Health

One thing that always shocks first-time airline passengers (at least, the first time you're old enough to understand the flight attendants' instructions) is that if there's a loss of cabin pressure, put the drop-down oxygen mask on yourself first, and *then* put your child's mask on the child. Not the other way around.

Similarly, one of the most interesting things about having a chronic condition like MS is that it forces you to prioritize, and it strangely makes you feel empowered to prioritize your own health more than you ever have before. You learn to say "no" to things that will get in the way of simply taking care of yourself; you have to assertively protect your downtime, your temperature, your sleep, your stress, and your food choices.

Otherwise, you can develop symptoms, which can range from numbness (which can cause partial paralysis) to vision problems (such as partial blindness or double vision) or walking problems. Following these recommendations listed in this chapter will help keep your condition mild and well under control.

Probably the strangest thing about this condition is that you can stay in the closet about it and never tell anyone. With modern medicine and the relatively new knowledge about managing the symptoms, someone may have MS and you'd never know it.

...Unless they're trying to bring a dozen Snack-Packs with them on the plane!

CHAPTER 2: ACHIEVING HEALTHY BODY CHEMISTRY

(Oh, great. Another MS diet. No thanks.)

Don't worry, this isn't an MS diet! I'm only going to focus on several basic, main strategies here to help keep us happy and healthy.

The book *Eat Right 4 Your Type* explains how each of the four blood types reacts (or doesn't) with various foods under a microscope, and how various foods are tolerated in the body of someone with each type. Dr. D'Adamo analyzed every single food with each of the four blood types: O, A, B, and AB.

Many foods didn't react at all with some or

all blood types under the microscope, and other foods reacted horribly with one or more types – making the blood cells agglutinate, or coalesce.

When this happens, the blood cells fasten to each other and combine into a mass, and a mass like this can interrupt normal bodily processes. It can be especially harmful if the agglutinated blood passes through the protective blood-brain barrier.

And in MS, it's of utmost importance to protect the brain.

The reactions under the microscope between the blood types and foods relate to why more than one human blood type exists in the first place. As people migrated into new areas, their bodies had to adjust to the new climates and new foods in order to survive:

- **First was Type O**, the hunter/gatherer, and they still do best on a diet of meats and vegetables that are fairly pure and unprocessed. Type Os tend to have stomach problems (including ulcers) because they eat what "everyone else" is eating, including foods that create a pH imbalance for themselves – such as milk or orange juice. They also tend to have a high rate of developing celiac disease.

Type Os tend to be attracted to high-energy, highly social things, but be aware of what causes stress for you. If you're a Type O, do your best to keep your stress levels under control, otherwise you're susceptible to cancers and digestive issues.

Type Os enjoy the longest lifespans in general of all four types, and I believe that that's because this type has had the longest amount of time in which to get the proverbial nicks out – biologically speaking – since it was first. Type O cells have had longer to adjust.

- **Second was Type A**, which developed during the Agrarian Society period of human development. Type As still do best on a vegetarian diet, and they also metabolize chicken, turkey, and most fish very well. But they don't do very well with eating red meats.

Just like their farmer ancestors, Type As prefer one-on-one interactions rather than participating in large groups, and they do best with focused, relatively calm activities and professions. They tend to love to teach!

In my experience, most people who fiercely proclaim that "everyone" should be vegetarian are Type As. (Type Os who are vegetarian tend to be out of balance. As an animal lover myself, I appreciate their rationale.)

- **Third was Type B**, which developed as humans migrated into the cold mountains. They started herding and domesticating animals and drinking their milk. Type Bs still digest milk products the most efficiently of the four types. They usually love milk.

But strangely, as this type evolved, these humans lost their ability to metabolize chicken well – and Type Bs still should try to stay away from eating chicken, although the eggs are fine. Eggs don't have the harmful lectins found in the muscle of chicken which agglutinate Type B blood.

As a Type B myself, the two foods I avoid like the plague are chicken and tomato. I happily substitute turkey or beef for myself. And bring on the pasta with alfredo sauce! No more marinara, ketchup, or drumsticks.

If my workplace is having a pizza party, they order a white pizza so I can participate. White pizza has no tomato sauce.

In my experience, Type Bs do better digesting processed foods than do Types O and A. Milkshakes and highly processed lunch meats don't usually give Type Bs a stomach ache like it can to others.

- **Fourth was Type AB**, which only occurs one person at a time – when the baby inherits a Type A gene from one parent and a Type B gene from the other – which is why it's the rarest of the four types. There is no "AB gene" to pass along.

  They do best on a combination of the A and B diets, but should mostly lean toward the Type A foods.

"So what?" Well, you might be regularly eating a food or two that are creating toxins in your body. And that same food doesn't necessarily create toxins in the body of someone with a different blood type than you.

Blood Type and MS

All of that helps to explain why there isn't a good "MS regimen" whose exact list of foods and exercises produces a beneficial reaction for everyone with MS.

Instead, the Blood Type Diet (and its related

blood-type recommendations, including supplements and types of exercise) involves eating the same foods, and moving (exercising) in the same ways, as when your own blood type was developing and evolving in human history. Dare I call them your "cellular ancestors"?

However, if your doctor has given you different dietary recommendations because of a certain health situation you have, please ignore the recommendations given here. Even if you have MS, you may have another condition that takes precedence.

Below are the key recommendations per your own blood type:

Type O:

- Eat plenty of red meat, chicken, turkey, and vegetables

- Eat salty snacks to satiate your palate

- Avoid corn and wheat like the plague

- Also avoid cow's milk and white potato (these aren't as dire)

- Engage in high-intensity exercises that push your muscles

Type A:

- Eat plenty of chicken, turkey, fish, fruits, nuts, yogurt, and vegetables

- Eat sweet and/or sour snacks to satiate your palate

- Avoid red meat and highly processed foods like the plague

- Also avoid cow's milk and shellfish (these aren't as dire)

- Engage in mild, calming exercises

Type B:

- Eat plenty of coldwater fish, beef, turkey, potatoes, and milk

- Eat dark chocolate or almond snacks to satiate your palate

- Avoid chicken and tomato like the plague

- Also avoid corn and shellfish (these aren't as dire)

- Engage in low-impact exercises

Type AB:

- Eat plenty of fish, turkey, vegetables, and cheese

- Eat peanut butter and nut-based snacks to satiate your palate

- Avoid chicken and beef like the plague

- Also avoid vinegar and corn (these aren't as dire)

- Engage in low-impact and calming exercises

It's my experience that most people don't know what blood type they have, and it can be hard to find out this information from your doctor. Whenever I've brought up this fact with a doctor, they always say something to the effect of, "Well, you don't need to know."

And that's true, insofar as they're concerned. If you're in a bad accident and need a quick transfusion, the hospital will give you Type O-negative blood, because they don't have time to test your type. And no one's body will reject O-negative blood.

Think of "O-negative" as literally "zero-nothing." There are no elements in O-negative blood that will have an adverse reaction with other blood types, because it doesn't have Type A's or Type B's sugar antigen on its blood cells. The Rh (positive/negative) component is the presence or lack of a protein antigen, and your body won't react to something that's not there (Rh-negative).

Finding Out Your Blood Type

Websites where you can buy an at-home blood-testing kit, so a friend or family member can test your type, include **BodyRedesigning.com** and **4YourType.com**. The test is not expensive, and you'll know your type in about

10 minutes.

Tip: Be sure not to use too much water in the test, or the results will be diluted and possibly inaccurate. Only use a small drop each. Also, when I test someone's type, I do the finger-prick in the thumb, as it's usually less painful than in the other fingers. Don't test someone who has frail skin or a blood disorder.

In figuring out which blood type can give and/or receive to others, I like to describe the compatibility of blood types like this:

O = Clear

A = Red

B = Blue

AB = Purple

...So thinking of the types in that way, you know who can give and receive to others, because you need to maintain your color and not ruin it.

Clear is acceptable to everyone, so clear can

donate to everyone. But clear can only receive clear. Purple can receive from everyone, but purple can only donate to other purple! Red can only receive red or clear; red can only donate to red or purple. Likewise with blue: receive blue or clear, donate to blue or purple.

Also for fun, think of positive/negative with the analogy of salt. If you're Rh-negative, you have no salt; Rh-positive has salt. (Again, this is only an analogy.) Salty can therefore accept unsalty, because it won't be ruined; but unsalty will be ruined by salty.

But as far as the Blood Type Diet goes, positive/negative doesn't matter.

You can find foods that are good for you at any restaurant. The preparation of the food isn't what's important; the food itself is what's important. For example, if beef is good for you but chicken isn't, it's actually better for you to have a greasy hamburger than broiled chicken breast.

When I started the diet 21 years ago, I felt like I was eating the way I liked to eat when I was little. I hope you do, too.

Thank You, Slim-Fast!

Here's how I found the Blood Type Diet:

About a year after my first "official" symptom – which was an episode of blinding optic neuritis in my left eye for five months – I was at work and was drinking a Slim-Fast, trying to lose a few pounds. A co-worker saw the shake on my desk and walked into my office.

"You should try the body-type diet," she said. "You eat based on your body type."

Well, heck, I was a child of the '70s and '80s, so I was always game for a new diet. (I still do love Slim-Fast shakes.) Cynthia remembered that the last name of the author started with "A," but she couldn't remember the full name. That was in January 1998, so we couldn't just Google it back then.

The A-Ha Moment...

The next day, I went to Waldenbooks to get the book Cynthia told me about. A young woman working there tried to help me look for this book in the Diets section. We looked at all the names of the authors, too.

"This one looks close to what you're looking for," she said, as she handed me *Eat Right 4 Your Type* by Dr. Peter D'Adamo. We both figured perhaps Cynthia meant the last name was D'A, because this book was about eating according to your blood type, so it certainly seemed similar.

The back of the book said things that were surprisingly accurate for me as someone with the B blood type. So I bought it.

Cynthia said it wasn't the book she'd told me about, but she glanced over the summary and said that it's very similar to her book.

I couldn't believe what this book was saying. First of all, it says that people with the B blood type like me tend to be better at fending off most cancers and heart disease than the other three types (O, A, and AB), but we tend to be susceptible to autoimmune conditions like MS, lupus, and Lou Gehrig's disease.

Wow! I'd had optic neuritis only a year earlier and was warned that I "might" have MS, so I was amazed that my blood type could be an explanation for all of this.

Incidentally, in the following months, I learned more and more relatives' blood types, and I found out that both of my grandfathers were Type A-negative, which is a very rare type. Most of my relatives are Type Os, As, and ABs, so their body chemistries are different than mine. No wonder it's not in my family!

I hope research is done to find out whether people with MS who are Type O or Type A had an ancestor who was Type B. Just a thought.

Eating Only What I Love

I was baffled to realize that the book was essentially telling me to go back to eating the way I used to like to eat when I was little: hamburgers, steak, turkey, milk, strawberries, grapes, pears, green beans, rice cereals, chocolate, etc. As I got older, I learned to eat the cultural diet – the foods everyone else was eating but which I didn't always enjoy.

Wow. Wow, wow wow. As I looked through the food lists, it all made sense. The science and logic behind it made me look forward to trying this diet out.

But I knew this would be a major change, too. Pasta marinara with chicken was one of my staples! I had to re-train myself, at least on this trial basis to see if this diet worked.

Cold-Turkey

My weekday lunch habit had always been to go to Taco Bell and get a soft taco and a bean burrito. So I called the headquarters of Taco Bell (again, this was before the Internet had everything!) and asked the customer service agent what the ingredients were in my burrito and taco.

Everything in the soft taco was fine for me.

"What kind of beans are in the bean burrito?" I asked.

"Pinto beans," she said.

I checked my Blood Type B list.

Ugh. Sure enough, pinto beans are on my Avoid list. Goodness! What was I going to have for lunch now?

I now wonder why I didn't just continue my "run for the border" lunchtime habit and just have four or five soft tacos, but I suppose I would have felt like I was really missing out on my bean burrito.

Day One

I plowed right ahead and started the diet the next day. It was January 15, 1998, and I was 26. That was during what I call "the innocent days of the Internet" because people would send emails to each other and forward jokes and self-executable files (.exe) that would play fun cartoons and stuff. Coca-Cola even sent out an email blast with an .exe file that gave you a "free cupholder for the holidays," and opening the .exe file would make your CD drive pop open! It was a clever, cute, fun joke.

One of the emails I received every day was a devotional Scripture passage, and on that day, the verse was Luke 14:33, which says that if you are not willing to "give up everything" then you cannot be His disciple.

How apropos! I was giving up "everything" all right.

But maybe I'll lose five pounds, we'll see.

During the first days on the diet, I had to get used to this whole new way of eating, and it felt good – I didn't feel deprived at all. I started to grab pita salad-sandwiches or order burgers without ketchup. I'd pick off every bit of tomato from all pre-made salads, even the slimy little seeds.

And the Healing Begins

After being on this diet for about two weeks, I was walking up the stairs into work one day and immediately noticed that my knees didn't hurt like they always did while using the stairs.

Must be the warmer weather, I figured. (The diet didn't even occur to me.) We were having an unseasonably warm spell there in the North Carolina winter, as it was about 70 degrees outside. My knees didn't hurt the next day, either, but it was still warm outside.

Two days later, it was getting cold again, but my knees didn't start hurting again while walking up those stairs. Waaaait a second...

It must be this strange diet! I thought. I wasn't absolutely sure, but as the days went on and my knees remained happy and ache-free, I became more and more sure.

I'd had those achy knees whenever ascending or descending stairs and hills probably since high school, or at least early college. It started so gradually that I didn't even notice.

Not Just Better Knees

I soon realized that the constantly dry skin on my hands had cleared up, too. I had developed the habit of applying moisturizer on my hands after washing them, because otherwise I'd have these awful cracks on my skin that would bleed – even though I was only 26. So the skin on my hands was back to normal, finally without cracks.

This was unbelievable! If just these two

outward signs – in my knees and my skin – were any indication of what might also be going on inside my body, this might be the healing I needed.

Little did I know that those foods on my Avoid list in the Blood Type Diet were causing so much damage to my body all those years. Well, thank God I found out now rather than later, when more damage could have been done.

But it turned out that I hadn't had the whole MS thing beaten quite yet. There was one more thing that had to be added to my repertoire.

CHAPTER 3: DX: MS –
AND MODERN MEDICINE

I was waking up on a bright and sunny Saturday in October 2000, now living in South Florida, and Ron and I were going to meet my sister Heidi's boyfriend for the first time that afternoon. As I got out of bed, I immediately noticed that the top half of my left thumb was numb.

I shook my hand, hoping that maybe I'd just slept on it or something and it was asleep. But the numbness wasn't going away.

Oh no, I thought. *Perish the thought that*

this could be an MS symptom.

But it was hard to perish the thought. It had been four years since the optic neuritis, which was when the ophthalmologist said that I might feel some tingling in my leg in five years.

I'd been strictly avoiding chicken, tomato, shellfish, pig meats, and everything else on the blood Type B's Avoid list for almost three years, seemingly "giving up everything" as the Bible verse said.

Advice I'd Been Ignoring

But I hadn't been as conscientious as I should have about avoiding hot showers and baths, which the National Multiple Sclerosis Society had recommended before.

The master bathroom in our new house had a Whirlpool tub. I had to take advantage of having this piece of luxury!

But I should have been as strict with the

water temperature as I'd been with the food, because only a week before this numb thumb, I'd taken a hot bath in that new tub.

My parents and Ron and I had fun having lunch together with Heidi and her boyfriend that afternoon at The Cheesecake Factory. Meanwhile, the numbness seemed to be creeping up my arm as the day went on – I tried to ignore it. That night when I took a shower, the water droplets felt uncomfortable hitting my left arm. It felt like someone was throwing little needles or tiny pellets at me.

The next morning, the numbness was definitely creeping further, because my whole left thumb was now numb, and the rest of that hand felt very tingly. That evening in the shower, the water droplets almost seemed to hurt my arm. I angled my body so the water would hit my right side instead.

The next day was a Monday, and I called and made an appointment with a neurologist whose office was near my workplace. He could see me on Thursday afternoon.

Wednesday evening before Ron came home from work, our bichon Mustard (think "Dijon mustard") was sitting on my lap as I searched online to see if I could figure out my condition before seeing the doctor the next day.

I went to the National MS Society's website. It was terribly humbling, but informative. The home page clearly listed the three most common first symptoms: optic neuritis, numbness, and walking problems.

Optic neuritis: Check. Numbness: Check.

Yep. I started to quietly cry. I knew what the doctor was going to tell me the next day. It hadn't taken a full five years for "tingling in your leg" and that ilk to show up. It had only been four years.

Mustard was a very intuitive little dog, and she immediately sat up on my lap and licked away my tears. I was so thankful to have her.

I figured I'd probably better get used to having this new scarlet letter, or two, attached to me – M-S.

Dx-Day

The next day, I left work early in the afternoon to go to my neurologist appointment. (And I was going back to work afterward, as if I were just getting my teeth cleaned or something.) The waiting room was fairly crowded. A young woman limped to the front after her name was called – she was tall and pretty, she seemed like the kind of girl who would have been in my ZTA sorority at the University of Florida. *Hmmm, I'm probably about to join her ranks, she probably has MS*, I thought.

Once my name was called, the nurse brought me to a room and told me to change into one of those paper outfits, open in the back. (I've since learned that *good* brain doctors let you keep your regular clothes on!) As the neurologist came into the room, he was like a tall grandfather, and he asked me what I was there for. He had a fairly thick foreign accent.

"I have this bad numbness in my left side," I said. I explained how it started in my left thumb and just kept spreading up my arm and to my neck/chest area. I said that I went on the Web and saw that optic neuritis and numbness are two of the major indicators of MS.

"So I know I probably have MS, because I had optic neuritis four years ago." I hoped that would speed things up.

Nope. I might have just made things worse. It was almost like he was the type who didn't want some non-doctor to tell him what to think.

He noticed that the outer edge of my left eye was constantly twitching. "Ah!" he said. "Let me show the nurse – she has had that, too!"

He got the nurse and she looked at my eye.

She smiled and nodded approvingly at me and at him. "See?!" he said almost gleefully to her.

The nurse left the room, and I asked him if she has MS.

"Oh! I can't tell you that!" he said.

(Great – thanks! He's lucky I was only 29, because today I would have confronted him about his unprofessional behavior. I'm not a specimen to be studied like a frog.)

He had me do all sorts of silly things (which seem normal after you've had a condition like MS for a while, because every neurologist does the same sort of movement-tests), and he asked me to go into the hallway so he could evaluate how well I walk.

As I was about to walk into the hallway, he acted surprised and said, "Oh! You're going to flash everybody!" And he wrapped another paper outfit around my back. (Hasn't he been doing this his whole career? Why the surprise?)

He had me walk up and down the little hallway, which I now know is one of the things every neurologist has an MS patient do during pretty much every visit.

The Tackiest MS Diagnosis Ever

Once we were back in the examination room, the wall-phone rang, and he answered it.

"Oh yeah! Are we going to play golf this Saturday? ... A ha ha! Yeah!"

I thought that was rude, but whatever. He had me do some more movement-tests, and the phone rang again. Same thing, but a different friend.

"Ah yeah! We're playing golf on Saturday, are you joining us? ...Ha ha! See you then!"

(Seriously? What am I, chopped liver?)

After hanging up with his pal, he turned to me and said in his accent, "You're just going to have to accept the fact that you have the MS."

Accept the fact?! I thought. That's how I get diagnosed – how totally tacky. He didn't even acknowledge that I was correct in my assumptions. On the contrary, he was acting like I was in denial. Sheesh!

"Okay," he said as he pointed at me. "Only do eight hours of work, eight hours of sleep, and eight hours of rest. Don't work any more than 40 hours per week. And don't agree to volunteer for things anymore. No more stress."

"So when am I supposed to exercise?" I asked.

He hesitated, as if he'd never realized before that his directive seems a bit contrary to his additional directive to get enough exercise.

"Well, during the 'rest' part," he said.

I'm actually glad he was the one to diagnose me, because his order to start saying "no" to things turned out to be a big help – very empowering. I'd been ignoring how much stress

I was feeling. And indeed, after saying "no" to volunteer requests for a while, I was able to slowly figure out which things I could agree to do, without pushing myself too much.

He then had me do some painful test for what seemed like an hour, literally testing my nerves. A couple of my fingers were hooked up to some machine, and a woman was asleep who was hooked up to the other machine next to me – which seemed strange. How do you sleep through this zapping?

A New Normal

After the appointment, I went back to work. It was only about 3:30 in the afternoon. But it struck me how everything seemed so normal – the traffic, the weather, the people – but my life was suddenly very un-normal.

My manager, Diane, came up to me at my desk and asked what I'd found out. (I had told her before my appointment that I was expecting to be diagnosed with MS.)

"Yeah, I do have MS," I told her. It felt like acknowledging some sort of defeat.

"Hmm. [Pause.] I once participated in an MS bike-a-thon fund-raiser!" she said with a smile, trying to make me feel better.

I smiled. "Thanks," I said, feeling strange that suddenly bike-a-thons like that were for people like me.

I called my parents that evening to let them know it was official. Ron and I had been looking into adopting a child, and Dad mentioned that and said, "You might want to hold off on that." It made me a little angry that this whole MS issue was interfering with so many things, but I knew he was probably right.

It also made me angry that my friends would now think of me as their "friend with MS." I'd remembered hearing black people on TV verbalize annoyance that their white friends think of them as "their black friend." They didn't want their color to be the defining thing. I totally could relate to that. It's angering because there's nothing noble you can do about it. (I eventually learned that rising above it, and not letting others' reactions bother me, was the best solution.)

The following day was a Friday, and the numbness became almost unbearably uncomfortable. It felt like a big monster was standing on my left shoulder – and it felt like if you put a pin into my left arm, blood would come gushing out like a fire hydrant – it was this enormous pressure. (The feeling is actually due to nerves, not actual pressure.) I noticed that it wasn't painful per se, just terribly uncomfortable, like a too-tight hug that you wish would stop!

I left work early and called the doctor's office. He prescribed a six-day regimen of a steroid, prednisolone. (A *steroid*?! Ugh.)

A Bright Spot

Some people who are diagnosed with MS have horrible fears of it at first, and they don't know anyone who has it. But I did.

I contacted the two people I knew who had MS. One was a woman from church, Sandy Kelley, and I talked to her on the phone. I also sent an email to *Boca Raton* magazine, because back in college I'd interviewed the co-owner of the magazine, John Shuff, so I could write a paper about how the magazine was founded.

An Officer and a Gentleman

John Shuff had told me back then that he was diagnosed with MS in 1975, and he kept working hard and was chief financial officer of Capital Cities (ABC) in New York City. So in 1981, after his condition had worsened, he and his wife, Margaret Mary, decided to pull up stakes and move to Florida for a more relaxed lifestyle.

They decided to use their skills and expertise

to start *Boca Raton* magazine, and so Margaret Mary did all the legwork while he directed.

I thought I was so clever as I entitled my college paper, "From Fighting Irish to Fighting Illness: The History of Boca Raton Magazine." (John Shuff is an alumnus of Notre Dame.)

So when I emailed his magazine after being diagnosed with MS, I said I'd like to talk with John Shuff since we now had this odd connection – and I mentioned that I'd interviewed him about seven years earlier. Only a couple days after I sent it, I received a wonderful voicemail from John Shuff! He gave me a little pep talk and told me the name of his neurologist.

I'll always feel indebted to Sandy and John for their important encouragement during that discouraging time. There's something to be said about getting feedback from someone who actually has the same condition you have.

Special thanks again to John for writing the foreword to this book. What a gentleman.

The Big Creep

Every day during this period of numbness, for several weeks, the numbness would creep further – first from my left thumb up my left arm, then up the left side of my neck and head, and then down the left side of my torso, down my left leg... Every day the creep would be further along. When would it stop? Would my whole body turn numb??

The numbness in my left hand got so bad that I temporarily lost my dexterity. I couldn't type very well with that hand for about six weeks; I'd use those fingers almost like sticks as I'd type, mostly the thumb and pinky. But I couldn't feel sensation, only pressure.

The numbness kept creeping (and not subsiding), eventually spreading to two middle toes on my right foot. Ugh – my right side now.

Then it jumped only to the tips of my middle and ring finger of my right hand.

And the spreading stopped.

The Medication

It stopped spreading exactly a week after I had my first shot of Avonex medication. The interferon beta 1-a isn't supposed to affect your current MS exacerbation, but it's hard not to attribute the sudden halt to the medicine at least a little.

A nurse had come to my house to give me the first injection of Avonex about two weeks after I was diagnosed. (I'd also had an MRI for further confirmation.) The shot only had to be done once a week, so she came to my house every week to give me the injection – I didn't want to do it myself.

Fortunately, before the first shot, the neurologist had told me that the injection is done in the outside of the upper leg, into the muscle. So I told the nurse I'd put on shorts for the injection, and I sat down on my barstool.

She said flatly, "Oh no, this one goes in the butt."

I said, "No, it can also go in the upper leg!" She looked at the flimsy paper pamphlet that came with the medication, and she agreed.

Ugh! That was close.

The nurse would alternate which leg would get the injection every week – right leg one week, left the next – to give the area "a break" between injections. It didn't even hurt, really. Not at first. I couldn't watch her while she did it, but it didn't bother me otherwise.

The nurse came every week for four months to give me the shot. In the fifth month, she said gently, "Your insurance company isn't going to keep covering me to give you your shot. Can I show your husband how to do it?"

"No, you can show me how to do it!" I said, smiling. She kept coming for another couple weeks to supervise me while I gave myself the injection. I was actually lucky that my insurance company paid her for those five months in 2000–2001, because I've heard that they're not as generous nowadays.

The needle part was about an inch long, and the injection went all the way in, into the muscle. She showed me how to do the shot, and it wasn't as difficult as I thought it would be. I'd write down which leg the shot was in every week so I wouldn't accidentally do it two weeks in a row in the same leg.

I eventually developed a way to give myself the shot: I'd put the tip of the needle very gently against my skin, and if it felt sensitive in the slightest, I'd move to a slightly different site and do the same thing. I could usually find a spot where it wouldn't hurt too badly. And I'd put the needle in verrrry slowly; once it was fully in, I'd push the plunger down very slowly as well. That usually worked very well and kept the pain to a minimum.

I was on that same medication for almost 16 year. The only reason I switched after 16 years was because those areas on my upper legs had become pretty hardened from basically being "stabbed" by the shot for all those years, and it was becoming painful. My new medication is the same type of medicine made by the same company, but (1) it has a longer-lasting, time-release formula, and (2) it's subcutaneous (under the skin) rather than intramuscular.

So I only have to do the shot once every two weeks now, which is nice. It's a pen-style injection like you see in the ads.

I think that, if I were diagnosed with MS right now, I'd opt for one of the oral medications. However, the issue with the oral medications is that all of them – as of the time of this writing – have had some users experience fatal side effects, namely PML (progressive multifocal leukoencephalopathy). Hopefully that will be resolved soon. I have a feeling it will.

Incidentally, a month after I was diagnosed, I told my nurse that I wanted to switch to a different neurologist. She recommended Dr. Feinberg – and he's been my neurologist for the past 18 years. He recently said to me, "I think you're probably my healthiest patient." (Yey!)

So even though many people tout avoiding medication and going the natural route, in my experience it's vitally important to be on one of the MS medications *in addition to* following the holistic and dietary methods, as described here.

Strict as I was, the dietary and lifestyle modifications didn't prevent me from being diagnosed with MS. Traditional medication helps to prevent flare-ups, disability, and the spread of the hidden disease process in the nervous system. And I'm thankful for it.

CHAPTER 4: HOW THE SYSTEMS BEGAN

Sorry for going back to the beginning here, but this book is designed to help you with your own MS – I'm the guinea pig, but I'm not the focus here, you are. So I didn't want to start out talking about my optic neuritis episode. Still, I'd like to explain how the SYSTEMS started in the first place. Now that I've explained the total solution, I'll tell you the first part of my story in case you're interested.

I couldn't tell which eye the "dot" was in.

It was a beautiful day in Cary, North Carolina – September 1996 – a normal Monday at work. I suddenly noticed when I looked away from my computer screen that there was a tiny dot in the middle of my vision. I looked up and down and all around, and closed my eyes to try to get rid of the dot. I even walked down the hallway and looked out the huge windows along the way – to give my eyes some exercise.

But the dot was still there! I couldn't even figure out which eye the dot was in. I tried covering each eye, but I couldn't tell. I closed my eyes for about 10 seconds to see if that would fix it. But it didn't.

How am I going to work with this annoying dot in my vision? I thought. *And what the heck is causing this?*

I was a technical editor at an IBM affiliate, so I had to be able to distinguish typos and small details. The dot was so distracting, both physically and psychologically.

But I plowed ahead and just tried to ignore it. I didn't even tell anyone at work that day – what would they say? It's not a common complaint for a 25-year-old woman to suddenly have a little fixed blind spot in her vision.

The day before, my (late) husband Ron and I had returned from visiting his Mom in New Jersey, and it wasn't until years later that I'd put two and two together: The water in the shower at her house was very hot, and I had a hard time adjusting the temperature without making it too cold – so I'd taken very hot showers during my entire visit there. (We had also moved from Florida to North Carolina within the previous year, complete with a new job and everything, so it had been a very stressful year.)

In retrospect, after I'd turned off the lights to go to bed on that Sunday night – the night after flying back home, and the night before this "dot" day – I'd noticed a flurry of stars in my vision against the dark room. Hmm.

So when I woke up the day after "dot" day, on Tuesday morning, the dot was larger. And now I could tell it was in my left eye. The dot was larger and larger every day, and meanwhile I was getting brief headaches that would come and go for no reason. I'm not even a "headache" person! Now it was getting scary.

Brain Cancer??

My maternal grandfather died of brain cancer when he was only 30, in 1947, when my Mom was 7 years old – and I was very aware that this could be it. I tried not to think about that. Perish the thought.

But the dot kept getting larger – creating an ever-increasing blind spot – and the headaches were becoming more frequent and more painful. Especially whenever I would move my eyes upward, I'd get an excruciating headache. I'd move my whole head upward so I wouldn't have to move my eyes upward very much.

Sinus Infection?

I was starting to tell a few people about the blind spot and the headaches, and one co-worker said it's probably a sinus infection.

Oh good! So I quickly made an appointment with my ear-nose-throat doctor, and I saw him that afternoon.

Nope. He didn't see any issues. Darn.

Headaches. Increasing partial blindness. It was really stressing me out to think that this could be my grandfather's brain cancer.

After a week of this, I realized I had to see an eye doctor to find out what in the world was happening.

Unscheduled Visit with the Doctor

So, very early on Monday morning, I went to my optometrist's office as soon as it opened. He was the only doctor in the practice who was there, so he gave me a once-over and handed me a bottle of eye drops. It was early in the morning, so none of the ophthalmologists were there yet to offer another opinion even if he'd wanted it.

"My roommate in college had this same thing," Dr. Bryan said. He didn't say what it was, but he did say it would probably go away. He pulled out a little pad whose pages each had a pre-printed grid with a dot in the center, and he ripped off the top page and handed it to me.

He told me to put it on the refrigerator so I could keep track of the progression of my vision changes. He said to cover my right eye, look at the dot in the center of the Amsler Grid, and pay attention to how much of the grid I could see with my left eye. And to do the same with the other eye so I could also see the difference.

The Amsler Grid was helpful but disturbing. I was losing the center of my vision in my left eye, but my peripheral vision stayed intact. The drops didn't help.

I went back there two days later to see an ophthalmologist at the practice, and Dr. Board examined my left eye – and he seemed almost agitated. It was obviously an uncommon thing to diagnose, even for an eye doctor.

"I wonder if that's optic neuritis," he said. "Let me get another doctor and get her opinion."

He soon came back into the room with another doctor, and she peered into my left eye.

"Do you think that's optic neuritis?" he asked her.

"Yes, I really think so," she said. She gave me a reassuring smile.

Dr. Board ordered an MRI of my brain. The most vivid memory I have from that day is of telling my parents on the phone later that night that I had to have an MRI. I was expecting them to be glad to hear that "next steps" were progressing, but they sounded worried. I was surprised, because they were usually so calm and tended to brush off things as handle-able.

But we all knew what happened to my grandfather. "Hopefully it's not a brain tumor," I said. It felt chilling just to verbalize it. They seemed relieved that I was the one to bring it up – they didn't want to.

Serious Tests Now

A couple days later, I went in to have the MRI. I'd decided beforehand to keep my eyes closed while they rolled me into the MRI machine and while inside it, because I'd seen it on TV before (everyone has!) and I knew it would make me feel claustrophobic.

So I was proud of myself as I kept my eyes closed while they put me into the MRI scanner, and I pictured myself sleeping in my bedroom, with the ceiling far above my head... But after a while, my curiosity got the best of me.

I opened my eyes just slightly – OOPS! Bad

idea! I instantly closed my eyes again and tried to picture being in my bedroom again, with the ceiling high above me!

Good News – and Possibly Bad News

Several days later, it was about 3 o'clock in the afternoon and I was at work, and Dr. Board called.

"Well, we got your MRI results," he said in his mildly Southern accent. "The good news is that there's no brain tumor."

"Oh, thank God!" I said, honestly thanking God. But I was very aware that he'd said "the good news" as a probable precursor to bad.

"But the thing is," he said, "optic neuritis can be a symptom of multiple sclerosis. Five years from now, you might have some tingling in your leg."

"Oh," was all I could muster. But inside I was thinking, *What??* MS isn't in my family –

this news was far out of left field.

"But your vision will most likely return back to normal after a while," he explained. He didn't say how long "a while" would be, but it did give me some hope amid this strange news of MS.

Dr. Board told me that I should bring the MRI films to a neurologist to find out what to do next, if anything. *A neurologist? Who has a neurologist?* I thought. Nobody my age, that I knew of.

I thanked him and hung up. Then I emailed my manager what I'd just heard, and I told her I was leaving for the afternoon because "I'm pretty shaken." I remember feeling strange typing that. It was as if I were saying it about someone else.

Start Spreading the News

I went home and put my little dog, Mustard, on my lap and called my parents. My Dad was actually home, so I told him everything the same way Dr. Board had told me. I said it's not a tumor, and he had the same three seconds of happiness and relief that I'd had. Then I told him it might be MS, and he was thrown off just like I was.

Still, MS is better than brain cancer, and we both knew that, even though we didn't know what else to really think. Ron was on a business trip, so my sweet little Mustard gave me lots of fluffy comfort that day.

Trying to mentally grasp this news was really odd. First thoughts, of course, were *Why?* I have a very large extended family – my parents each have seven siblings, and almost all of those siblings have two or more children – and none of my aunts or uncles or cousins have MS. The family has various cases of addictions and cancers, but not MS or anything like it.

I started being overly aware of everything that is abbreviated as "MS" or has the word "multiple" in it. Microsoft. Mississippi. MSNBC.

MS Word. Massanetta Springs. Ms. MS-13. Master of science. Multiple births, multiple ownership, multiple copies, multiple personalities. ...

The Wishy-Washy Neurologist Appointment

So several days later, Ron and I went to see a neurologist. The doctor looked at my MRI films and quickly saw a few small spots on a couple of the films. He even took his ballpoint pen and circled the spots. (I was surprised he wrote right on them without asking me first!)

"I'd expect to see these results from an MRI of *your* brain [pointing to Ron, who was 24 years older than me], but not hers."

We kept asking him if it was MS, but he hemmed and hawed. "What's the *percentage* of a chance that it's MS?" we asked.

"Sixty percent," he said.

Well, that wasn't very much help. I really wanted to put a name on this – this *thing*.

"We'll have to wait and see whether you get a second symptom, and it would have to be different than optic neuritis for an MS diagnosis. And then we'd put you on a medication," he explained.

If Only I'd Remembered...

And here's where I later wished I'd remembered something that happened only two years earlier, so I could have told this neurologist about it. I realized it several years later, when I was searching through my daily journals to find out when exactly Ron and I went on a dinner cruise from Fort Lauderdale.

I'd written in a December 1994 entry: "My right leg has been numb for the past 4 days."

I couldn't believe I'd totally forgotten about that!

If I would have remembered that my leg had been numb for four days two years earlier, the neurologist might have diagnosed me with MS right then and there. But during those four days when my leg was numb (at age 23), my co-workers said it was "probably just a pinched nerve," so I dismissed it.

Most of us with MS have experienced this, with others dismissing numbness as a symptom of a pinched nerve or other fleeting malady.

Slowly Blinded, then Slowly Sighted Again

During this episode of optic neuritis, the headaches abruptly went away after exactly two weeks. The blind spot in my left eye kept getting larger and larger in the center of my vision, then remained large for about two or three months. Then it gradually improved, and my sight fully returned to normal when it was over – five months after it started.

I happened to find out just the year before

from Dr. Bryan that my left eye was actually my dominant eye, so I was aware that my right eye had "taken over" during those five months. So as my left eye took over again, I experienced really strange visual effects, which made driving pretty crazy! The trees on both sides of my car (in my peripheral vision) seemed to "stagger" as I drove past them. Like a jerky motion, or as if there were really old movies playing on both sides of my car.

Pirate Eye

As the optic neuritis was improving, I went to a costume store and bought a pirate's eye patch, and I wore it over my right eye whenever I was padding around the house. That way, I figured it would help force my left eye to be dominant again. It was pretty annoying having two eyes trying to be dominant, so it was a relief to wear the eye patch – and I think it actually worked pretty well.

I was just glad my vision was finally getting

better again. In the meantime, Ron called the National Multiple Sclerosis Society, and the girl on the phone told him that I should avoid taking hot showers and baths. It didn't occur to me until much later that the shower water at his Mom's house in New Jersey had been so hot during our visit.

Reading My First Publication Acceptance with One Eye

The really neat thing that happened during that period of optic neuritis was receiving my first letter of acceptance from a publisher. It was from Broadman & Holman Publishers, accepting my three-year Bible-reading plan! I remember having to re-read the letter over and over again just to make sure this was really happening!

The Lord has a cool way of uplifting us when we're at a low moment in life, doesn't He.

CHAPTER 5: SYMPTOMS ALL ALONG, IN RETROSPECT

As it turns out, those four days of numbness in my right leg at age 23 may not have been my first MS symptom after all. In retrospect, there were several precursors that may have indicated an underlying health issue.

Prior Illnesses and Conditions

Researchers say that many people with MS have slow-growing viruses which were acquired years before developing MS. Similarly, a website I saw soon after my diagnosis alluded to a possible correlation between the streptococcal bacterium and MS. (A bacterial infection is different from a viral infection, but they can cause similar problems.)

The bacterial point hit home. I'll start there:

- **Scarlet fever and strep throat at age 6.** It was Christmas Day 1977 – and my family had recently moved from Bellaire, Ohio, to Minneapolis, Minnesota – when it got really bad. Christmas fell on a Sunday that year, and my Dad is a (now retired) Presbyterian minister; so Mom and my sister, Heidi, stayed home with me while Dad went to church. When he got home, he brought me to the Minneapolis Children's Hospital, where I was quickly diagnosed with both strep throat and scarlet fever. They're caused by the streptococcal bacterium. (My pediatrician had said it was just a cold.)

  I'm blessed to have had scarlet fever in

the 1970s rather than, say, the 1870s, because the Minneapolis Children's Hospital prescribed the antibiotic ampicillin, and I was fine within 10 days. Ampicillin is a mild form of penicillin that fights bacteria – in my case, streptococcal bacteria. People used to die or go blind from scarlet fever.

I remember church people visiting me at home and whispering as they spoke to me. I wondered why they were all whispering.

A number of years later, I told my Mom that I'd wondered why everyone was whispering to me when I had scarlet fever, and she said, "Actually, they were all *yelling* so you could hear them."

- **Breaking my leg at age 7.** This may or may not have been an MS precursor, but a broken bone may indicate a susceptibility or weakness when assessed collectively with the other things.

All we wanted to do was to get out of the house so my Dad could enjoy watching his Pittsburgh Steelers in the Super Bowl that afternoon (this was January 21, 1979). My Mom took Heidi, our friend Amy, and me to go ice-skating at a nearby rink for the afternoon. I broke my leg only about a minute after getting onto the rink! I was trying to do a backwards leg-lift like Dorothy Hamill in the 1976 Olympics, but I literally fell flat. I heard a snap and everything.

Dad came to the rink and took me to the Minneapolis Children's Hospital. He saw the Steelers win the game on a little black-and-white TV in the waiting room! (Hey, at least they won.)

You could argue that it's normal for a child to break a leg, but kids do crazy things all the time and they don't break their legs that easily.

- **All of those days in high school and college when I was drop-dead tired.** I often barely had the energy to get out of bed. You may say this is normal, too, but there was no reason for it. A doctor diagnosed me with "depression" twice in high school – I actually missed 25 days of school in my senior year.

   I now wonder if many of those days were during football season, because I was in the marching band and we'd have long practices in the Florida heat.

   And in college, I remember the housemom at my sorority driving me to the school's infirmary (student clinic), and I was expecting to be diagnosed with mono. But the diagnosis was vague, and they gave me some basic medicine to help with the fatigue.

- **Mildly achy knees when ascending and descending stairs and hills,**

probably since high school. This was a symptom that developed gradually over many years. I ignored it and didn't even give it much thought until it suddenly went away in January 1998 after I started the Blood Type Diet. It was very, very obvious when the pain wasn't there anymore.

- **Having to sit down while taking a morning shower in college.** I was a sophomore at the University of Florida in 1990 when five students were murdered in their Gainesville apartments. The killer was on the loose, so I went home to West Palm Beach and transferred to Florida Atlantic University in Boca Raton for the semester. The Florida universities did a wonderful thing by extending their registration period so UF students could transfer, and not miss a whole semester.

But all the daytime classes were taken

at FAU, so I had to take nighttime classes. I've always taken a shower at night before bed, so this reversed my normal routine – and I'd take a shower in the morning so I wouldn't keep my parents awake at night.

But several mornings during my shower, I'd suddenly feel lightheaded and I'd have to sit down on the ledge. That was weird.

What I realized is that I'd first have to eat something cold for breakfast – like cereal – before my shower, not after. Otherwise I'd feel faint like that.

For more than two decades now, my habit has been to drink Carnation Instant Breakfast (now called Breakfast Essentials) with milk practically every single morning. It's a cold drink and has lots of nutrition, and I think it's ideal for those of us in the, uh, Mu Sigma society. Especially those of us with Type B blood.

Each of these things individually isn't necessarily a precursor of MS, but collectively they can paint a broader picture.

When a woman at my church asked us on the Deacons board to pray for her teenage son because he was having tests for some unusual health issues, I thought about the fact that she is Type B (which she'd told me), and I figured he might be Type B as well.

So I asked her if her son had ever had scarlet fever. Her reaction was similar to that of the woman at Walgreens: first no, and then, well, actually, yes.

She already knew I have MS, and I told her my story and I explained that he might eventually develop it – and that it's a very manageable condition if he does. People don't usually realize that it's better to have MS than other conditions which display similar symptoms!

CHAPTER 6: LET THEM EAT CHOCOLATE!

My Mom likes to tell people about the time when I was 5 years old, and she asked me what I wanted to do when I grew up.

"I want to write a book," I said.

After hearing myself say that, I was suddenly inspired to go ahead and do just that! Why wait? So I took a little notepad and wrote a book (or, short story) called "Sroop." Sroop was a happy little alien who lived on the planet Waksee. Waksee was made entirely of chocolate, and it had "all the vitamins and minerals" necessary for survival! (I was such a child of the 1970s, concerned about "vitamins and minerals" at age 5.)

But after a while, because all the inhabitants of Waksee ate only Waksee itself, the planet was getting too small to hold everyone.

They needed help!

So Sroop had an idea – he wrote a note asking for help, put it in a bottle, and threw it up into the sky.

Soon, a spaceship came bringing lots of food for all the people of Waksee! So Sroop was the hero.

The Visceral Need for/Love of Chocolate

So, obviously, I've always loved chocolate – it was almost like a need, not a want. But my parents didn't want my sister and me to get cavities, so we didn't eat it very often. I didn't like dark chocolate back then, but I always loved M&M's and Hershey's milk chocolates.

I remember reading a little book about 1976

Olympic gymnast Nadia Comaneci playing soccer with her friends back in Romania, and they'd "play for chocolate bars." Mmm, chocolate bars! It sounded so delectable!

I loved doing gymnastics in our living room and everywhere else (I wanted to be the next Nadia), and yet even with all that exercise, I always had a problem with my (ahem) constitution. I don't get stomach aches like many people do, but I've always had constant issues with my plumbing.

And from reading various publications and websites, this is a fairly common issue for those of us with MS.

I've discovered that eating pure dark chocolate every day is a delicious solution to this problem, at least for me.

Dentists have told me that pure chocolate is actually a preferred snack food over crunchy or sticky snacks, because chocolate rinses out of the teeth easily.

The Christmas Blessing

The women of Trinity Presbyterian Church in Raleigh, North Carolina, celebrated at a special Christmas get-together at Diane Keely's house in 1999. She had a vast assortment of sweets and treats for all of us to enjoy.

One candy dish had individually wrapped Dove milk chocolates in blue foil and dark chocolates in red foil. I sampled a milk chocolate one, and even though I didn't really like dark chocolate, I tried a dark chocolate one.

Woah! I could almost sense that this wonderful treat was actually good for me. Not the eating-too-many-Doritos sort of good (as in, can't my life just be a continuous munch-a-thon on these?!), but good in a nutritious sort of way.

Daily Chocolate

So after this revelation of a love for dark chocolate, I started consuming Dove dark chocolates at work every day. I soon realized that my (ahem) constitution was working so much better!

It was all coming together now – even back when I wrote "Sroop" at age 5, I must have been craving chocolate to balance out my system.

Dark chocolate is so rich that I don't overeat it. I've even realized that I now like all brands of dark chocolate, including Hershey's, Ghirardelli, and Lindt. I even like the really dark stuff, like semisweet and baker's chocolate.

In fact, with my new dark-chocolate weekday consumption, I discovered something. On the weekends when I wouldn't eat any chocolate, my personal plumbing issues would come back. And they'd be fixed again on Monday after eating some chocolate.

Who knew?

Chocolate Helps Solve One MS Problem

Even though this solution brings balance to my body, it won't have the same effect on everyone, of course. But I would argue that those of us with MS should try it (unless you're allergic), because there is a tendency for digestive issues among those of us with MS – and it's obviously related to maintaining a healthy gut.

(Always beware of health nuts who don't have MS trying to tell you what to eat and what not to. MS puts us in a whole different category that doesn't follow the rules.)

I've found that I need to have at least six individually wrapped, bite-size dark chocolates each day for my body to process foods properly. The fact that they're individually wrapped makes it easier to control the portion size – if I'm deep in thought at work, I usually don't feel like stopping to unwrap a chocolate.

I've learned not to deviate from pure dark chocolate, though! If the chocolate has almonds, I'll eat too many of them. The variety increases the cravings, whereas a constant diet of the same pure dark chocolate every day helps to prevent overindulging.

If You Can't Have Chocolate...

If you're allergic to chocolate or you don't like it, choose a favorite snackable food on your "Beneficial" or "Neutral" list from the Blood Type Diet and enjoy it every day. Oatmeal and oat bars, and almonds and almond bars are a good option. Yum!

CHAPTER 7: WHY?
BLAME THE VIKINGS (SORT OF)

In the spots around the world where the ancient Vikings stopped to plunder and pillage, there are much higher incidences of MS than in other areas of the globe. Hmm!

This phenomenon has been studied thoroughly, and PBS even created a documentary about it entitled "Multiple Sclerosis, the Vikings and Nordic Skiing," originally aired in 2013. This factoid brings some logic to the odd distribution of MS, because otherwise the patterns are broken – just a smattering here and there.

And since we're giving some credence to the blood-type connection with MS, the Viking factor might also help to explain why the countries in Asia and the Middle East (where Type B appears in the highest percentages) have *lower* incidences of MS than those in northern Europe and Britain. After all, the Vikings spent much more time in northern Europe and the surrounding region than anywhere else.

Scotland consistently ranks as having one of the highest prevalence rates of MS, and the Vikings spent a lot of time there and largely settled there. Most of the people I know who have MS do have some Scottish ancestry.

The Viking theory also intrigues me because of the fact that heat can exacerbate MS symptoms. The Vikings thrived in cold climates; the early people with the B blood type also thrived in cold climates. Hmm.

Theories About Regions of the World

When you're diagnosed with something like MS, you're hungry for any piece of information you can find about the condition. Soon after I was diagnosed, one of the statistics I kept seeing was about people who moved to a different region before or after age 14.

If you moved from a "high-risk region" (where there's a higher incidence of MS) to a low-risk region before age 14, then you're more likely to mirror the MS tendency of your new region. But if you moved after age 14, you keep your original tendency from the place where you moved from.

Since my family moved from Minneapolis, Minnesota, to West Palm Beach, Florida, several months after my 14th birthday, this statistic was true for me! My body did keep my original high-risk tendency from Minnesota.

And the Vikings are Minnesota's team!

Or the Vitamin D Connection?

Much of the research about who gets MS around the world focuses on the fact that MS is more prevalent in regions where people have low amounts of exposure to the sun, and therefore low amounts of natural vitamin D absorption.

However, I can't help but think of this as a chicken-and-egg theory – whiter people tend to have less vitamin D absorption, and whiter people tend to get MS more than darker people. So, which came first? Do the low vitamin D levels cause (or aggravate) MS susceptibility, or do the inherited genes (not related to vitamin D) cause the susceptibility?

I'm not convinced that low amounts of sun exposure has a causative effect, but the jury is still out! Stay tuned.

Don't Blame Artificial Sweeteners

I don't know if this rumor got started by an organization or company that was trying to stir up distrust and negative opinions about artificial sweeteners, but don't listen to the artificial sweetener–MS connection rumor. Using a normal amount of artificial sweeteners (such as aspartame and saccharin) in your coffee or tea has nothing to do with your risk of developing MS.

However, people whose bodies have difficulty digesting processed foods may do best using regular, pure sugar and honey.

Beware of people who have a singular solution or a monofaceted theory about MS. They obviously don't understand the complexities of MS. They're probably just trying to sell you something!

CHAPTER 8: THE TAKEAWAY

I once attended a day-long seminar about church growth, and the seminar happened to be held at my own church. The leader gave us some really good ideas and input, and it all seemed straightforward and simple enough to implement – and very exciting!

The leader said, "Now, most of your churches won't make ANY of these changes in order for your own church to grow!"

That shocked me, especially since it seemed like his ideas and recommendations would be easy to do.

But he was right. My church didn't make any of the changes, and we hosted the seminar! And sure enough, we've had difficulty growing because people are naturally resistant to even minor changes.

It can be hard to make a change, even when it's relatively simple to implement. Just because something is simple doesn't mean it's easy.

Rah-Rah!

With this in mind, remember that you're completely in control of your own body. You now have some great ideas from this book to try for yourself, and see if they help improve your MS. Perhaps they'll help improve things you didn't even realize could be improved.

If you strictly (yes, strictly!) follow these recommendations – as long as your doctor doesn't give you a good reason not to – you should start to notice improvements to your health in about three weeks.

As far as the "E" (Eat Right) factor goes, remember that avoiding the foods that are bad for you will likely make a big difference in your health. Try not to rationalize that it's "only a little" or "just this time," such as putting ketchup on a hamburger if tomato is bad for you, or having a burger if beef is bad for you.

I promise you, you'll be able to find alternatives that you naturally prefer anyway.

You will do best to **avoid these ingredients** if you are:

- **Type O**: Avoid corn and wheat
- **Type A**: Avoid red meat and highly processed foods
- **Type B**: Avoid chicken meat* and tomato
- **Type AB**: Avoid beef and chicken meat*

* Chicken eggs are fine; avoid anything that involves chicken meat, including broth.

And whatever your blood type, enjoy a dose of pure dark chocolate (or your alternate of choice) every day to keep your constitution healthy – to keep your digestion working fully, from top to bottom.

If you're having trouble getting the medication your doctor prescribes, call the manufacturer of the medicine directly. Pharmaceutical companies have received a bad rap, but they do want to help. Give them that opportunity.

Finally, go to church and thank the Lord you live in a time and place where you have everything you need to address this health challenge. Before MRI technology, they would just give you a hot bath and wait to see if you'd have a reaction. Yeah. Thanks for today, Lord.

Your Unwanted Promotion!

The thing about having MS is that your friends, relatives, and associates will have a whole new perspective of you, so you're in the spotlight now – whether you want to be or not. In what seems like a backwards way, you have the opportunity to be a leader of sorts. Show them how to handle adversity with grace, joy, and self-control.

You can't control others, but you can control yourself, and you can be an example for them to follow. They're watching you closely and curiously. Smile!

In fact, this brings us full-circle back to the entire context of the "thorn in the flesh" illustration:

"Therefore, so that I would not exalt myself, a thorn in the flesh was given to me, a messenger of Satan to torment me so I would not exalt myself. Concerning this, I pleaded with the Lord three times to take it away from me.

"But He said to me, 'My grace is sufficient for you, for power is perfected in weakness.' Therefore, I will most gladly boast all the more about my weaknesses, so that Christ's power may reside in me."

~ II Corinthians 12:7-9 (CSB)

Aim for the Arrest

I've heard my MS described as a "complete arrest of the disease process" and "inactive." Who knew "arrest" and "inactive" could be such beautiful, beautiful words!

Two years after my MS article was published in Newsmax, I happened to drive by the woman from Walgreens, who was riding her scooter-chair on the sidewalk. I actually had a printout of the article in my car, so I stopped and reintroduced myself, and gave her the article! That was on August 26, 2010 – exactly two years to the day of publication.

I wanted to write this book so that you don't have to just figure it out on your own. I believe God has shown me the method – the SYSTEMS – for controlling my MS. Join me in living life to the fullest!

> **"…but our God turned the curse into a blessing."**
>
> **~ Nehemiah 13:2 (HCSB)**

BIBLIOGRAPHY AND
RECOMMENDED READING

NewsmaxHealth.com, "Defeating MS: From Curse to Blessing," Heather Collins Grattan, Copyright © August 26, 2008.

Eat Right 4 Your Type: The Individualized Diet Solution to Staying Healthy, Living Longer and Achieving Your Ideal Weight, Dr. Peter J. D'Adamo with Catherine Whitney, G.P. Putnam's Sons, Copyright © 1996.

ABOUT THE WRITERS

Heather Collins-Grattan Floyd is the author of *The Compatibility Matrix: The Qualities of YOUR Ideal Mate, An Open Letter to Charles Krauthammer,* and *Trump in the Middle: Why America Needs a Middle Child This Time Around.* She devised the 3-year Bible-reading plan for the *HCSB/CSB Study Bible,* and she was a contributing writer to *Nelson's New Christian Dictionary.*

Mrs. Floyd was diagnosed with MS in 2000. She holds a bachelor's degree in journalism from the University of Florida, and she is an active Presbyterian elder and deacon. She lives in Florida with her husband, Kevin, and their pit-bull and bichon frisé, Jigsaw and Ketchup.

John Shuff is the co-founder and owner of JES Publishing, which produces *Boca* magazine, *Delray* magazine, *Salt Lake* magazine, *Worth Avenue,* and *Mizner's Dream.* He also writes a column entitled "My Turn" for the magazines.

Mr. Shuff was diagnosed with MS in 1975. He founded JES with his wife, Margaret Mary. They live in Florida.

Made in United States
Orlando, FL
12 April 2022